New and Emerging Areas in Medicine Series

Telehealth Competencies Across the Learning Continuum

Association of American Medical Colleges
Washington, D.C.

The AAMC (Association of American Medical Colleges) is a not-for-profit association dedicated to transforming health through medical education, health care, medical research, and community collaborations. Its members are all 155 accredited U.S. and 17 accredited Canadian medical schools; more than 400 teaching hospitals and health systems, including Department of Veterans Affairs medical centers; and more than 70 academic societies. Through these institutions and organizations, the AAMC leads and serves America's medical schools and teaching hospitals and their more than 179,000 full-time faculty members, 92,000 medical students, 140,000 resident physicians, and 60,000 graduate students and postdoctoral researchers in the biomedical sciences. Additional information about the AAMC is available at aamc.org.

Suggested citation: AAMC. *Telehealth Competencies Across the Learning Continuum.* AAMC New and Emerging Areas in Medicine Series. Washington, DC: AAMC; 2021.

ISBN: 978-1-57754-197-4

AAMC

Contents

Preface

Health care is changing rapidly. New technologies, advances in care delivery, and scientific discoveries are happening at rates that make it challenging for teaching and learning practices across the continuum to keep up. Whether learners are at the beginning of their career or seasoned clinicians, new demands and advances in health care require them to acquire new competencies. The AAMC New and Emerging Areas in Medicine Series is a guide for everyone who develops curricula within the field of medicine and for people learning to practice or continuing their professional development.

Each set of new and emerging competencies is developed by leaders from across the medical education and clinical practice communities, including hundreds of reactors who review iterative drafts. The new competencies are intended to supplement existing ones (e.g., entrustable professional activities and milestones). These competencies add depth to selected emerging areas to help guide curricular and professional development, formative performance assessment, cross-continuum collaborations, and, ultimately, improvements in health care services and outcomes. This series also includes competencies in quality improvement and patient safety (aamc.org/what-we-do/mission-areas/medical-education/cbme/qips), and competencies in diversity, equity, and inclusion are in development. The competencies are not intended for high-stakes assessment or for purposes of accreditation.

Acknowledgments

The AAMC acknowledges the dedication of the talented members of the Telehealth Advisory Committee, who helped develop and revise draft competencies, and the hundreds of students, residents, faculty, affiliates, patient advocates, and others who reviewed drafts throughout the iterative development process. We thank them for their dedication to advancing telehealth through education and collaboration across the continuum.

Telehealth Advisory Committee, 2019-2020

Andrea Borondy Kitts, MS, MPH
Patient Outreach and Research Specialist
Lahey Hospital and Medical Center

Shruti Chandra, MD, MEHP
Clerkship Director, Emergency Medicine
Sidney Kimmel Medical College at Thomas Jefferson University

Neil Evans, MD
Chief Officer, Connected Care
Veterans Health Administration

Kevin Galpin, MD
Executive Director, Telehealth Services
Veterans Health Administration

Emily Hayden, MD, MHPE
Director of Telemedicine
Massachusetts General Hospital

Kristi Henderson, DNP, NP-BC, FAAN, FAEN
Senior Vice President, Innovation and Telehealth
Optum Health
University of Texas at Austin Dell Medical School

Toyia James-Stevenson, MD
Medical Director for GI Access, GI Quality and Women's GI Health
Indiana University Health

Elizabeth A. Krupinski, PhD, FSPIE, FSIIM, SATA, FAIMBE
Professor and Vice Chair for Research
Department of Radiology and Imaging Sciences
Emory University

Joseph Kvedar, MD
Senior Advisor of Virtual Care and Professor of Dermatology
Mass General Brigham and Harvard Medical School

David Lambert, MD
Senior Associate Dean for Medical Student Education
University of Rochester School of Medicine and Dentistry

Chen-Tan "CT" Lin MD, FACP, FAMIA
Chief Medical Information Officer
UCHealth, Colorado

Curtis Lowery, MD
Director of the Institute for Digital Health and Innovation (IDHI)
University of Arkansas for Medical Sciences

James Marcin, MD, MPH
Director, Center for Health and Technology, and Professor of Pediatric Critical Care
UC Davis Children's Hospital, UC Davis Health

Karen S. Rheuban, MD
Medical Director, Office of Telemedicine
Senior Associate Dean for Continuing Medical Education and External Affairs
University of Virginia

Ariel Santos, MD, MPH, FACS, FCCM
Director of Telemedicine, Chief of Acute Care Surgery
Texas Tech University Health Sciences Center

Neal Sikka, MD
Chief of the Innovative Practice and Telemedicine Section, and Professor of Emergency Medicine
GW Medical Faculty Associates

AAMC Staff

Adrien Barrios
Program Specialist, Strategic Initiatives and Partnerships in Medical Education

Sarah Hampton
Program Specialist, Clinical Innovations

Keith Horvath, MD
Senior Director, Clinical Transformation

Lisa Howley, PhD, MEd
Senior Director, Strategic Initiatives and Partnerships in Medical Education

Kate Ogden, MPH
Policy and Regulatory Analyst, Physician Payment and Quality

Janis Orlowski, MD, MACP
Chief Health Care Affairs Officer
Executive Co-Sponsor

Scott Shipman, MD, MPH
Director, Clinical Innovations

Kamilah Weems, MS
Director, Strategic Initiatives and Partnerships in Medical Education

Alison Whelan, MD
Chief Academic Officer
Executive Co-Sponsor

Series Introduction

Competency-based education (CBE) is a developing approach to health professions education. The AAMC has a long history with CBE and defining the fundamentals for practicing in an increasingly complex health care system. Over the past 20 years, medical education has improved in many ways, including in how outcomes such as competencies are defined and used to guide teaching and learning. To support this kind of positive change, we are offering the New and Emerging Areas in Medicine Series. The series frames competencies across the undergraduate, graduate, and continuing medical education continuum. This report includes an introduction to CBE, competencies in telehealth, and the importance of developing competence in this area, as well as tactics for integrating this essential educational focus into the curriculum. Details about the development process and a glossary of terms are included as appendixes.

CBE has its roots in primary education and psychology, and its use in medical and other health professions education has grown significantly since the late 1990s. Around that time, the AAMC introduced the Medical School Objectives Project,[1] and the Accreditation Council for Graduate Medical Education (ACGME) and the American Board of Medical Specialties (ABMS) announced six general competency domains for physicians.[2] Before that, schools and programs had focused more on the processes of curricular or program administration and less on the performance outcomes of learners.

The significant shift from educational processes to outcomes led medical knowledge and patient care domains to expand to interpersonal communication, professionalism, practice-based learning and improvement, and systems-based practice. These six domains are now broadly adopted by other groups within and outside medicine and across the continuum of professional development. They are often a framework for developing a set of competencies, including the current set. A guiding question in developing competencies is, What does a physician, progressing toward attainment of expertise, do, know, and value in relation to the construct in question?

The Case for Telehealth Competencies

Telehealth, defined as the use of technology to deliver health care at a distance, has become an increasingly important and commonly used tool for delivering care to patients. Even before the COVID-19 pandemic, providers' use of telehealth in teaching hospitals was growing steadily.[3] To better understand the evolving role of telehealth, the AAMC hosted a meeting of national telehealth experts to discuss the opportunities and risks for telehealth for academic medicine in 2016. The message from participants was clear: If telehealth were to be useful in the provision of high-quality care and be adopted by clinicians in a generalizable and sustainable way, providing training in telehealth to the clinician workforce would be essential. To guide a path forward, a set of consensus physician competencies in telehealth was needed. To address this need, the AAMC established a Telehealth Advisory Committee tasked with first identifying the skills needed by physicians to provide high-quality care via telehealth, independent of setting or specialty.[4] Once the skills were identified, the committee brought in additional experts in education to help translate the skills into competencies for each stage of the medical education continuum. COVID-19 intensified the need for these competencies. They will provide a foundation of support to ensure medical schools and teaching hospitals are providing excellent training to physicians and other clinicians in all forms of telehealth.

Organization of the Competencies and Intended Uses

Organization

These competencies were developed over 18 months through an iterative process that began with Telehealth Advisory Committee members working together to articulate the set of skills required by clinicians to provide high-quality care via telehealth, independent of specialty or setting. Those skills were modified further and, with extensive stakeholder feedback, translated into competencies (refer to Appendix A for details). The competencies are organized into six domains: 1) Patient Safety and Appropriate Use of Telehealth, 2) Access and Equity in Telehealth, 3) Communication via Telehealth, 4) Data Collection and Assessment via Telehealth, 5) Technology for Telehealth, and 6) Ethical Practices and Legal Requirements for Telehealth — and three tiers that represent developmental stages in physician development: 1) entry to residency or recent medical school graduate, 2) entry to practice or recent residency graduate, and 3) experienced faculty physician or three to five years post-residency.

Intended Uses

These cross-continuum competencies are intended to help educators design and deliver curricula and related activities and to help learners in their individual professional development in telehealth. The cross-continuum competencies supplement existing competencies (e.g., entrustable professional activities and milestones) with more detail or depth; guide telehealth curricular and professional development, formative performance assessments, and cross-continuum collaborations; and, ultimately, improve health care services and outcomes. They are not intended to be used for high-stakes assessments or accreditation of schools, programs, or institutions. They are for use in:

- Engaging diverse health care professionals in collaborative telehealth discussions, including cross-continuum and cross-discipline colleagues.
- Conducting gap analyses of local curricula and training programs.
- Planning individual professional development.
- Developing curricular learning objectives.
- Developing assessment tools.
- Furthering research and scholarship in medical education and telehealth.
- Guiding the strategic integration of telehealth into the curricula and the clinical learning environment.

Telehealth Competencies

Health care is changing rapidly. New technologies, advances in care delivery, and scientific discoveries are happening at rates that make it challenging for teaching and learning practices across the continuum to keep up. Whether learners are at the beginning of their career or seasoned clinicians, new demands and advances in health care require them to acquire new competencies. The AAMC New and Emerging Areas in Medicine Series is a guide for everyone who develops curricula within the field of medicine and for people learning to practice or continuing their professional development.

Domain I: Patient Safety and Appropriate Use of Telehealth

Clinicians will understand when and why to use telehealth and how to assess patient readiness, patient safety, practice readiness, and end-user readiness (Table 1).

Table 1. Domain I: Patient Safety and Appropriate Use of Telehealth

Entering Residency **(Recent Medical School Graduate)**	**Entering Practice** **(Recent Residency Graduate)** *All Prior Competencies +*	**Experienced Faculty Physician** **(3-5 Years Post-Residency)** *All Prior Competencies +*
1a. Explains to patients and caregivers the uses, limitations, and benefits of telehealth — that is, the use of electronic communications technology to provide care at a distance	1b. Explains and adapts practice in the context of the limitations and benefits of telehealth	1c. Role models and teaches how to practice telehealth, mitigate risks of providing care at a distance, and assess methods for improvement
2a. Works with diverse patients and caregivers to determine patient and caregiver access to technology to incorporate telehealth into patient care during real or simulated encounters	2b. Works with diverse patients and caregivers to evaluate and remedy patient and practice barriers to incorporating telehealth into patient care (e.g., access to and comfort with technology)	2c. Role models and teaches how to partner with diverse patients and caregivers in the use of telehealth
3a. Explains to patients and caregivers the roles and responsibilities of team members in telehealth encounters regardless of modality	3b. Demonstrates understanding of all roles and works as a team member when practicing telehealth regardless of modality	3c. Coordinates, implements, and evaluates the effectiveness of the telehealth team regardless of modality
4a. Describes when patient safety is at risk, including when and how to escalate care during a telehealth encounter (e.g., converts to in-person visit or emergency response)	4b. Prepares for and escalates care when patient safety is at risk during a telehealth encounter (e.g., converts to in-person visit or emergency response)	4c. Role models and teaches how to assess patient safety during a telehealth encounter, including preparing for and escalating care when patient safety is at risk

Domain II: Access and Equity in Telehealth

To promote equitable access to care, clinicians will understand telehealth delivery that addresses and mitigates cultural biases as well as physician bias for or against telehealth and that accounts for physical and mental disabilities and non-health-related individual and community needs and limitations (Table 2).

Table 2. Domain II: Access and Equity in Telehealth

Entering Residency **(Recent Medical School Graduate)**	**Entering Practice** **(Recent Residency Graduate)** *All Prior Competencies +*	**Experienced Faculty Physician** **(3-5 Years Post-Residency)** *All Prior Competencies +*
1a. Describes one's own implicit and explicit biases and their implications when considering telehealth	1b. Describes and mitigates one's own implicit and explicit biases during telehealth encounters	1c. Role models and teaches how to recognize and mitigate biases during telehealth encounters
2a. Defines how telehealth can affect health equity and mitigate or amplify gaps in access to care	2b. Leverages technology to promote health equity and mitigate gaps in access to care	2c. Promotes and advocates the use of telehealth to promote health equity and access to care and to advocate for policy change in telehealth to reduce inequities
3a. When considering telehealth, assesses the patient's needs, preferences, access to, and potential cultural, social, physical, cognitive, and linguistic and other communication barriers to technology use	3b. When considering telehealth, accommodates the patient's needs, preferences, and potential cultural, social, physical, cognitive, and linguistic and communication barriers to technology use	3c. When considering telehealth, role models how to advocate for improved access to it and accommodates the patient's needs, preferences, and potential cultural, social, physical, cognitive, and linguistic and communication barriers to technology use

Domain III: Communication via Telehealth

Clinicians will effectively communicate with patients, families, caregivers, and health care team members using telehealth modalities (Table 3). They will also integrate both the transmission and receipt of information with the goal of effective knowledge transfer, professionalism, and understanding within a therapeutic relationship.

Table 3. Domain III: Communication via Telehealth

Entering Residency **(Recent Medical School Graduate)**	**Entering Practice** **(Recent Residency Graduate)** *All Prior Competencies +*	**Experienced Faculty Physician** **(3-5 Years Post-Residency)** *All Prior Competencies +*
1a. Develops an effective rapport with patients via real or simulated video visits, attending to eye contact, tone, body language, and nonverbal cues	1b. Develops an effective rapport with patients via video visits, attending to eye contact, tone, body language, and nonverbal cues	1c. Role models and teaches effective rapport-building with patients via video visits, attending to eye contact, tone, body language, and nonverbal cues
2a. Assesses the environment during real or simulated video visits, such as attending to disruptions related to privacy, lighting, sound, and attire	2b. Establishes therapeutic relationships and environments during video visits, such as attending to disruptions related to privacy, lighting, sound, and attire	2c. Role models effective therapeutic relationships and environments during telehealth encounters
3a. Explains how remote patients' social supports and health care providers can be incorporated into telehealth interactions and the care plan (e.g., asynchronous communication and the storage and forwarding of data)	3b. Determines situations in which patients' social supports and health care providers should be incorporated into telehealth interactions, with the patients' consent, to provide optimal care	3c. Role models and teaches how to incorporate patients' social supports into telehealth interactions, with the patients' consent, to provide optimal care

Domain IV: Data Collection and Assessment via Telehealth

Clinicians will obtain and manage clinical information via telehealth to ensure appropriate high-quality care (Table 4).

Table 4. Domain IV: Data Collection and Assessment via Telehealth

Entering Residency **(Recent Medical School Graduate)**	**Entering Practice** **(Recent Residency Graduate)** *All Prior Competencies +*	**Experienced Faculty Physician** **(3-5 Years Post-Residency)** *All Prior Competencies +*
1a. Obtains history (from patient, family, and/or caregiver) during a real or simulated telehealth encounter	1b. Obtains history (from patient, family, and/or caregiver) during a telehealth encounter and incorporates the information into differential diagnosis and the management plan	1c. Role models and teaches the skills required to obtain a history (from patient, family, and/or caregiver) during a telehealth encounter and incorporates the information into the management plan
2a. Conducts appropriate physical examination or collects relevant data on clinical status during a real or simulated telehealth encounter, including guiding the patient and/or tele-presenter	2b. Conducts appropriate physical examination and collects relevant data on clinical status during a telehealth encounter, including guiding the patient and/or tele-presenter	2c. Role models and teaches the skills required to perform a physical examination during a telehealth encounter, including guiding the patient and/or tele-presenter
3a. Explains the importance of patient-generated data in the clinical assessment and treatment plan during a telehealth encounter	3b. Incorporates patient-generated data into the clinical assessment and treatment plan while understanding data limitations and adapting accordingly	3c. Role models and teaches how to incorporate patient-generated data into the clinical assessment and treatment plan while understanding data limitations and adapting accordingly

Domain V: Technology for Telehealth

Clinicians will have basic knowledge of technology needed for the delivery of high-quality telehealth services (Table 5).

Table 5. Domain V: Technology for Telehealth

Entering Residency (Recent Medical School Graduate)	**Entering Practice (Recent Residency Graduate)** *All Prior Competencies +*	**Experienced Faculty Physician (3-5 Years Post-Residency)** *All Prior Competencies +*
1a. Explains equipment required for conducting care via telehealth at both originating and distant sites	1b. Identifies and is able to use the equipment needed for the intended service at both originating and distant sites	1c. Able to use, and teach others while using, equipment for the intended service at both originating and distant sites
2a. Explains limitations of and minimum requirements for local equipment, including common patient-owned devices	2b. Practices with a wide range of evidence-based technologies, including patient-owned devices, and understands limitations	2c. Role models and teaches how to incorporate emerging evidence-based technologies into practice, remaining responsive to the strengths and limitations of evolving applications of technology
3a. Explains the risk of technology failures and the need to respond to them	3b. Demonstrates how to troubleshoot basic technology failures and optimize settings with the technology being used	3c. Teaches others how to troubleshoot basic technology failures and optimize settings with the technology being used

Domain VI: Ethical Practices and Legal Requirements for Telehealth

Clinicians will understand the federal, state, and local facility practice requirements to meet the minimal standards to deliver health care via telehealth (Table 6). Clinicians will maintain patient privacy while minimizing risk to the clinician and patient during telehealth encounters, putting the patient's interest first, and preserving or enhancing the doctor-patient relationship.

Table 6. Domain VI: Ethical Practices and Legal Requirements for Telehealth

Entering Residency **(Recent Medical School Graduate)**	**Entering Practice** **(Recent Residency Graduate)** *All Prior Competencies +*	**Experienced Faculty Physician** **(3-5 Years Post-Residency)** *All Prior Competencies +*
1a. Describes locally relevant legal and privacy regulations for telehealth	1b. Complies with legal and privacy regulations for telehealth at the local, state, and federal levels	1c. Role models and complies with legal and privacy regulations for telehealth at the local, state, and federal levels
2a. Defines components of informed consent for the telehealth encounter	2b. Obtains informed consent for the telehealth encounter, including defining how privacy will be maintained	2c. Role models and teaches how to obtain informed consent for the telehealth encounter, including defining how privacy will be maintained
3a. Demonstrates knowledge of ethical challenges and professional requirements in telehealth	3b. Identifies and supports solutions that mitigate ethical problems and adhere to professional requirements in telehealth	3c. Identifies and seeks to address system-level solutions to ethical challenges that adhere to professional requirements in telehealth
4a. Describes potential conflicts of interests that may arise in the use of telehealth such as interest in commercial products or services	4b. Explains and discloses potential conflicts of interest to patients in the use of telehealth	4c. Explains and ensures all members of the care team disclose possible conflicts of interests in the use of telehealth

Curricular Models for Integrating and Improving Telehealth in Medical Education

This section includes profiles of telehealth curricula at a few member schools. The medical educators at these institutions serve on the AAMC Telehealth Advisory Committee and provided these summaries to demonstrate the many diverse and innovative approaches to teaching and learning about telehealth. MedEdPORTAL® is actively seeking submissions on telehealth education at mededportal.org.

University of Rochester School of Medicine and Dentistry
Double Helix Curriculum — Translations and Transitions Meliora in Medicine
David R. Lambert, MD
Senior Associate Dean for Medical Student Education

The longitudinal Rochester Meliora in Medicine telehealth curriculum traverses four phases, roughly correlating to four years of medical school. In the formative Phase 1, medical humanities faculty provide historical context about transitions in health care from the home to the hospital and back to the home. Foundational concepts, including the variety of telehealth modalities, are illustrated with local examples. In small groups, students discuss a telehealth case through different lenses, including access to care, continuity of care, cost, and interprofessional teams. Students are introduced to basic strategies for conducting a video visit and "webside manner." They view a live demonstration of a video visit and participate in a discussion with the physician, patient, and technician. A third session introduces patient-portal communication and confidentiality issues in communicating with adolescents.

Assessments include written exam questions, reflections, and response to a mock patient-portal query. In the Phase 1 assessment, students conduct telephone and video visits. In Phase 2, students complete three online modules and self-assessments, building on key telehealth concepts and providing more advanced guidance on conducting a video visit. A tipsheet organized by organ system provides tips for conducting physical exams on children and adults; students use the tipsheet during telehealth visits in their primary care clerkship. In their basic science courses, problem-based-learning cases illustrate how providers receive, evaluate, and act on data exchanged through telehealth modalities. In Phase 3, pediatrics clerkship students participate in a school-based telehealth experience. Finally, in Phase 4, specialty-specific telehealth topics, economics, and policy are introduced.

Sidney Kimmel Medical College at Thomas Jefferson University Telehealth Curriculum

Shruti Chandra, MD, MEHP
Program Director, Digital Health and Telehealth Education

At Sidney Kimmel Medical College, all medical students are trained in telehealth before they start their clinical rotations. The training, delivered through online modules and physical-exam videos, addresses the appropriate use of telehealth in different situations and its regulatory and legal aspects. Every clinical rotation has a plan to employ telehealth in some capacity, such as in outpatient visits, virtual rounding, callbacks, and tele-triage. Students perform visits under the supervision of faculty and receive summative and formative feedback on their telehealth skills.

Faculty perform a "bedside" evaluation of the student's skills with every visit, which allows them to assess history-taking skills, physical-examination techniques, professionalism, and interpersonal communication skills. This process also requires faculty development in how to supervise and assess students during a virtual visit with a patient. Additionally, all students have access to patients' electronic medical records, and visits are performed on a three-way platform. Lastly, telehealth is used as a tool for education and assessment through online virtual simulation, small-group and large-group lectures, and objective structured clinical examinations (OSCEs) and procedural-skills assessment.

Renaissance School of Medicine at Stony Brook University
Telehealth Education

Kimberly Noel, MD, MPH, Telehealth Director and Deputy Chief Medical Information Officer, Stony Brook Medicine
Erin Hulfish, MD, Director, Telemedicine Education, Renaissance School of Medicine, Stony Brook University

Stony Brook Telehealth offers a range of educational programs for undergraduates, graduate students, and clinicians. The Renaissance School of Medicine at Stony Brook University offers a mixed learning environment with traditional lectures and active learning with group discussions, self-directed reading exercises, and practicums. The preclinical courses, such as "Docs, Data and Disruptive Technologies," introduce telehealth practice as well as relevant laws, ethics, and regulations and the evolving doctor-patient relationship. The courses review current applications of telemedicine and future implications for the practice of medicine. Post-clinical telehealth courses are also offered, allowing students to have hands-on experience including communications training, "webside manner" training, and objective structured clinical examinations (OSCEs) in partnership with the Stony Brook Clinical Simulation Center. The courses also introduce new technologies for learning remote patient monitoring.

Telehealth education is promoted by Stony Brook's Interprofessional Telehealth Board, an academic collaborative of representatives from all five health science schools. The group creates educational resources for the community and develops standards for the practice of telehealth across disciplines, facilitates interprofessional research, creates and suggests interprofessional curricula, and explores interprofessional clinical experiences. The board creates curricula integrating the Interprofessional Education Collaborative (IPEC) competencies with the AAMC telehealth competencies to prepare the next generation for team-based virtual care. Stony Brook also trains resident physicians for the Tele-Preventive Medicine service (TPM) and trains preventive medicine residents to concurrently perform virtual visits focused on preventive care and, to optimize care, apply population health management methods and tools, including data analytics and quality improvement.

UC Davis Health
Telehealth Curriculum
James Marcin, MD, MPH, Professor, Pediatric Critical Care

UC Davis Health has a long history of using telehealth to improve patient care. Since its inception, the telehealth program has been integrated into care delivery and has provided real-time clinical services in nearly 50 pediatric and adult specialties. Through the Center for Health and Technology, UC Davis Health developed an internationally acclaimed telehealth and e-health curriculum for community-based health care providers and their patients. It has translated that experience into education and training for medical students, residents, and practicing physicians. With students in the early phases of their medical education, it works to impart the basic needs for any telehealth visit: establishing that the patient is comfortable with the video encounter, documenting that the identification process has been certified, and ensuring that the patient's wishes for the video visit are addressed.

The teaching and training emphasize key techniques for working within the telehealth environment to enable clinicians to remotely assess the objective nature of a patient's symptoms and physical signs. The telehealth platform used allows multi-person, simultaneous clinical visits so patients, care providers, translators, residents, and attending physicians can meet from different locations. It facilitates both the teaching and clinical workflows, enabling attending physicians to supervise and assess students and residents during telehealth encounters. UC Davis' telehealth curriculum was developed with an educational continuum in mind to expose health care providers to, train them in, and document their mastery of a variety of telehealth skills. That learning process provides students, residents, and practicing physicians with the skills and expertise necessary for successful telehealth care.

Appendix A. Development Process and Survey Questions

Development Process

There is no single standard approach to the development of competencies, but there are some preferred steps:

1. Define the scope of the competencies or the construct.
2. Engage diverse stakeholders and collect data to understand the nature of the construct. How do high performers perform? How do those who achieve positive results behave in practice? Gather data through literature reviews, focus groups, and electronic surveys of subject matter experts.
3. Draft the competencies.
4. Have reactor panels of subject matter experts, patients, frontline clinicians, and educators review multiple drafts of competencies.
5. Importantly, review and update competencies periodically to keep pace with changes in clinical and educational practices.

The telehealth competencies were translated from a set of telehealth skills for practicing physicians, so their development followed a slightly different process. In early 2019, the AAMC convened the Telehealth Advisory Committee to begin developing telehealth skills. The committee first met in person to review an AAMC-conducted literature review. Together, the committee drafted a set of domains that reflected results from the literature review and their own experience and expertise. Committee members then worked in teams to draft skills for each of the domain areas. Domains and skills were reviewed by the full committee and sent for stakeholder feedback, which was incorporated into the final set of domains and skills.

In late 2019, the Telehealth Advisory Committee added five medical educators with expertise in telehealth to the committee and convened in person to begin translating the telehealth skills into tiered competencies. Once the domains and competencies were drafted, we took several approaches to collecting stakeholder feedback. We collected feedback at the ACGME 2020 Annual Educational Conference, but due to the COVID-19 pandemic, we were unable to collect feedback through focus groups at AAMC meetings.

We used a modified Delphi method to further refine the competencies and increase stakeholder input. This included developing a questionnaire of standard items (refer to the Survey Questions on page 15), conducting iterative email rounds with that questionnaire, collecting individual or group feedback between rounds, and summarizing the findings. An electronic questionnaire inviting feedback about the initial domains and competencies was initially distributed to 326 stakeholders in April-May 2020. The stakeholders who received that questionnaire included people engaged in health professions education, research, and direct patient care and experts in telehealth.

We used the feedback from the first iteration to revise the domains and competencies and made multiple changes to the competencies across the three tiers and within all domains. The second questionnaire was sent in July 2020 to 335 stakeholders and included the same questions as the first version and a revised set of domains and competencies.

The response rates for the first and second surveys were 81% and 54%, respectively. We analyzed the mixed-methods data from the two surveys and further revised the competencies. Feedback from the first round of survey responses led to the grouping of two domains, Patient Safety and Appropriate Use of Telehealth, into one domain.

Overall, there was a slightly more favorable response to the second questionnaire, with an average score across all Likert scale items that was 4.5% higher in the second survey than in the first survey, indicating the competencies "will be helpful to them as they educate students, residents and/or physician faculty." We then shared the final draft of the telehealth domains and competencies again with the Expert Working Group for further refinement. The final version 1.0 of the telehealth competencies is on pages 4-9.

Survey Questions

Respondents, including focus group members and reactor panelists, reviewed the draft domains and related competencies and answered the following six standard questions about each domain:

1. *Importance: Does this set of draft competencies represent abilities that are important to high-quality, safe care? Response Options: 1 — No, not at all; 3 — Somewhat; 5 — Yes, definitely. Please describe your response:*

2. *Tier: Does this set of draft competencies reflect observable abilities at the appropriate level for entering resident (recent medical school graduate), entering practice (recent residency graduate), or experienced faculty physician (3-5 years post-residency)? Response Options: 1 — No, not at all; 3 — Somewhat; 5 — Yes, definitely. Please describe your response:*

3. *Comprehensive: Does this set of draft competencies reflect all specific abilities that are relevant to this domain? Response Options: 1 — Not at all; 3 — Somewhat; 5 — Yes, definitely. Please describe your response:*

4. *Granularity: Does the language reflect an optimal level of granularity? Response Options: 1 — No, not at all; 3 — Somewhat; 5 — Yes, definitely. Please describe your response:*

5. *Relevance: Do these competencies represent abilities that are relevant for all physicians regardless of their specialty and/or setting of practice? Response Options: 1 — No, not at all; 3 — Somewhat; 5 — Yes, definitely. Please describe your response:*

6. *Please provide general feedback on this subset of competencies:*

At the end of the questionnaire, respondents were asked to consider the full set of draft competencies in the six telehealth domains and answer four questions:

1. *What, if anything, is missing? (open-ended)*

2. *Do the six domains listed appropriately represent the breadth of telehealth? Please explain:*

3. *Do these draft competencies represent the depth of telehealth? Please explain:*

4. *How can we make these competencies most helpful? (open-ended)*

Appendix B. Glossary

care plan: "A written, personalised care plan, which, under the single-assessment process, details a patient's integrated health and social care needs."[5]

competency-based medical education: "An outcomes-based approach to the design, implementation, assessment, and evaluation of medical education programs, using an organizing framework of competencies."[6]

conflicts of interest (COI): Financial or other interests that may influence physicians in their roles with commercial health websites and services. Physicians must disclose COI and take active steps to manage or eliminate them.[7]

consensus: "Middle ground, between total assent and total disagreement."[1]

digital divide: The division between those who have access to and use information technology (typically, those who are younger, have higher education and income, and live in urban areas) and those who do not.[8]

e-consults: Asynchronous, consultative, provider-to-provider communications within a shared electronic health record (EHR) or web-based platform.[9]

ethical challenges unique to telehealth: Possible challenges to ensuring that telemedicine is ethically acceptable include erosion of the patient-doctor relationship, threats to patient privacy, forcing one-size-fits-all implementations, and the temptation to assume that new technology must be effective.[10]

experienced faculty physician: A person with an MD or DO degree who has completed residency and at least three years of independent practice and who teaches or supervises learners either paid or volunteer, full- or part-time.

explicit bias: "The traditional conceptualization of bias. With explicit bias, individuals are aware of their prejudices and attitudes toward certain groups. Positive or negative preferences for a particular group are conscious."[11]

health equity: The principle underlying a commitment to reduce — and, ultimately, eliminate — disparities in health and in its determinants, including social determinants.[12]

implicit bias: Also known as unconscious bias, refers to attitudes or stereotypes that are outside our awareness but nonetheless affect our understanding, our interactions, and our decisions.[13]

informed consent: "Permission obtained from a patient to perform a specific test or procedure. Informed consent is required before most invasive procedures are performed and before a patient is admitted to a research study."[14]

patient-generated data: Information recorded and gathered by patients, often through the use of technology such as smartphones and wearable devices.[15]

patient portal: A secure online website that gives patients convenient 24-hour access to personal health information from anywhere with an Internet connection.[16]

racial/ethnic bias: Refers to attitudes or stereotypes that affect our understanding, our interactions, and our decisions about race and ethnicity. The ways racial/ethnic bias can affect health range from limiting access to quality medical care and the physiological responses to the experience of chronic discrimination to inequitable exposures to occupational and environmental hazards.[17]

remote patient monitoring: Using digital technologies to collect medical and other forms of health data from individuals in one location and electronically transmit that information securely to health care providers in a different location for assessment and recommendations.[18]

role model: "One who serves as an example for others by demonstrating the behavior associated with a particular position or profession."[14]

simulated encounter: A technique (not a technology) to replace and amplify real experiences with guided ones, often immersive in nature, that evokes or replicates substantial aspects of the real world in a fully interactive fashion.[19]

telehealth: The use of electronic communications technology to provide care at a distance, including through patient portals, e-consults, video visits, and remote patient monitoring.

tele-presenter: "A medical professional at the originating site [who] presents a patient to the physician or practitioner at the distant site."[20]

therapeutic relationship: The relationship between a caregiver and a patient that includes the caregiver's valuing the patient, commitment to the patient, managing the power imbalance, and character and competencies.[21]

virtual visits: "Live, synchronous, interactive encounters between a patient and a healthcare provider via video, telephone, or live chat."[22]

References

1. Anderson MB, Cohen JJ, Hallock JE, Kassebaum DG, Turnbull J, Whitcomb M. *Report I: Learning Objectives for Medical Student Education — Guidelines for Medical Schools.* Washington, DC: AAMC; 1998.
2. Batalden P, Leach D, Swing S, Dreyfus H, Dreyfus S. General competencies and accreditation in graduate medical education: an antidote to overspecification in the education of medical specialists. *Health Aff.* 2002;21:103-111. https://geiselmed.dartmouth.edu/cfm/education/PDF/Article1.pdf. Accessed Aug. 8, 2019.
3. AAMC. AAMC Council of Teaching Hospitals Annual Survey of Hospital Operations and Financial (OpFin) Annual Report. https://www.aamc.org/data-reports/teaching-hospitals/report/opfin-report. Accessed September 2020.
4. Galpin K, Sikka N, King SL, et al. Expert consensus: telehealth skills for health care professionals [published online ahead of print Nov. 25, 2020]. *Telemed e-Health.* doi.org/10.1089/tmj.2020.0420.
5. Segen JC. *The Dictionary of Modern Medicine.* Park Ridge, NJ: Parthenon Publishing Group;1992.
6. Frank JR, Snell LS, Cate OT, et al. Competency-based medical education: theory to practice. *Med Teach.* 2010;32(8):638-645. doi:10.3109/0142159X.2010.501190.
7. Chaet D, Clearfield R, Sabin JE, Skimming K, on behalf of the American Medical Association Council on Ethical and Judicial Affairs. Ethical practice in telehealth and telemedicine. *J Gen Intern Med.* 2017;32(10):1136-1140. https://doi.org/10.1007/s11606-017-4082-2.
8. Connolly KK, Crosby ME. Examining e-health literacy and the digital divide in an underserved population in Hawai'i. *Hawai'i J Med Public Health.* 2014;73(2):44-48.
9. Vimalananda VG, Gupte G, Seraj SM, et al. Electronic consultations (e-consults) to improve access to specialty care: a systematic review and narrative synthesis. *J Telemed Telecare.* 21(6):323-330. https://doi.org/10.1177/1357633X15582108.
10. Mehta SJ. Medicine and Society: Telemedicine's Potential Ethical Pitfalls. *Virtual Mentor: AMA J Ethics.* 2014;16(12):1014-1017. doi:10.1001/virtualmentor.2014.16.12.msoc1-1412.
11. U.S. Department of Justice. Understanding Bias: A Resource Guide. Washington, DC: U.S. Department of Justice; 2015. https://www.justice.gov/crs/file/836431/download. Accessed Aug. 8, 2019.
12. Braveman P. What are health disparities and health equity? We need to be clear. *Public Health Rep.* 2014;129(Suppl 2):5-8. doi:10.1177/00333549141291S203.
13. Glicksman E. Unconscious bias in academic medicine: how the prejudices we don't know we have affect medical education, medical careers, and patient health. *AAMC Reporter.* 2017;January. https://www.aamc.org/news-insights/unconscious-bias-academic-medicine-overcoming-prejudices-we-don-t-know-we-have.
14. Myers T, ed. *Mosby's Medical Dictionary.* 8th ed. St. Louis, MO: Mosby Elsevier; 2009.

15. Department of Health and Human Services. What are patient-generated health data? HealthIT.gov. 2018;Jan. 19. https://www.healthit.gov/topic/otherhot-topics/what-are-patient-generated-health-data. Accessed Oct. 22, 2020.

16. Department of Health and Human Services. What is a patient portal? HealthIT.gov. 2017;Sept. 29. https://www.healthit.gov/faq/what-patient-portal. Accessed Oct. 22, 2020.

17. Cain VS, Kington RS. Investigating the role of racial/ethnic bias in health outcomes. *Am J Public Health.* 2003;93(2):191-192. doi:10.2105/ajph.93.2.191.

18. Atreja A, Francis S, Kurra S, Kabra R. Digital medicine and evolution of remote patient monitoring in cardiac electrophysiology: a state-of-the-art perspective. *Curr Treat Options Cardio Med.* 2019;21:92. https://doi.org/10.1007/s11936-019-0787-3.

19. Lateef F. Simulation-based learning: just like the real thing. *J Emerg Trauma Shock.* 2010;3(4):348–352. https://doi.org/10.4103/0974-2700.70743.

20. Telehealth Alliance of Oregon. Telepresenters. https://www.ortelehealth.org/content/telepresenters. Accessed September 2020.

21. Razzaghi, M.R, Afshar L. A conceptual model of physician-patient relationships: a qualitative study. *J Med Ethics Hist Med.* 2016;9:14.

22. American Telemedicine Association. Telehealth: Defining 21st Century Care. https://www.americantelemed.org/resource/why-telemedicine/. Accessed Nov. 20, 2020.

Made in the USA
Monee, IL
05 November 2026

67374693R00017